ESSEN

BEGINNERS

A BEGINNERS GUIDE TO NATURAL
HEALING AND AROMATHERAPY

By K. Connors

Table of Contents

INTRODUCTION 4

CHAPTER ONE 7

THE HISTORY OF ESSENTIAL OILS 7

CHAPTER TWO 16

WHAT ARE ESSENTIAL OILS? 16

CHAPTER THREE 28

WAYS OF PRODUCING ESSENTIAL OILS 28

CHAPTER FOUR 47

WHERE TO BUY ESSENTIAL OILS 47

CHAPTER FIVE 53

POPULAR OILS WITH HEALING PROPERTIES 53

CHAPTER SIX 60

AROMATHERAPY FOR PETS 60

CHAPTER SEVEN 66

ESSENTIAL OILS FOR CHILDREN 66

CHAPTER EIGHT 74

ESSENTIAL OIL DILUTION 74

CONCLUSION 77

INTRODUCTION

As common ingredients in natural products, essential oils are used commonly through inhalation or by topical application of diluted oil. Because these oils are so readily available to the public, many people incorrectly assume that no particular knowledge or training is needed to use them. Unfortunately, there are many who make this mistake. Some have read a little about aromatherapy, or a friend or supplier has told them a particular oil is good for this or that. But, essential oils can cause problems if used incorrectly. How much do you really know about these powerful botanicals?

Essential oils are chemical compounds with aromatic properties found in the seeds, roots, stems, bark, flowers, and other parts of plants. For centuries, there have been many stories of healing properties of these precious oils. There were also many ways essential oils were extracted out of different plants. For example, rose oil was extracted by massaging leaves with animal fat. A lot of essential oils, like Lemon and Orange, are cold pressed. The vast majority of oils from plants are steam distilled at a certain temperature and a specific pressure. The most therapeutic oils with optimum benefits are taken after the first distillation.

Topical use of essential oils is also very common and safe. The only controversial topic of topical use is a neat application. Neat application occurs when the essential oils are put directly on the skin without dilution. Many companies state that most of their oils are safe for neat application. Use caution when using oils in this way. Essential oils are VERY potent.

A single drop of oil is equal to seventy-five cups of tea with that particular plant. Such potency can be an issue with skin irritation. The most important rule with essential oils is to dilute them in carrier oils. Carrier oils are plant-based fatty oils used to dilute essential oils.

A good rule of thumb is to always perform a skin patch test using 1 drop of essential oil in 1ml of carrier oil. This creates a 5% solution. So, if you have 5ml carrier oil (or 1 teaspoon), 5 drops of essential oil is the maximum to maintain the 5% solution. There are many safe carrier oils like vegetable oil, coconut oil, sweet almond oil, grape seed oil, jojoba oil, olive oil, and other oils.

Internal use is the most controversial topic of aromatherapy. A lot of reputable companies endorse internal use; however, most Aromatherapy and Herbal Associations, including the International Federation of Aromatherapists (IFA) contraindicate the internal use of essential oils in their code of ethics by health care providers. The National Association of Holistic Aromatherapy discourages aromatherapists from using essential oils internally unless trained to do so. They are currently exploring the safety of internal use. So, contact a Certified Clinical Aromatherapist (CCA) for internal use.

CHAPTER ONE

THE HISTORY OF ESSENTIAL OILS

Essential oils were mankind's first medicine. From Egyptian hieroglyphics and Chinese manuscripts, we know that priests and physicians have been using essential oils for thousands of years.

Today, modern science is rediscovering the wisdom of the ancients. Essential oils are able to reach deep into the recesses of our brains, cross over the chemical barriers, and open the hidden channels within our minds and bodies. Essential oil fragrances pass on to the limbic system of the brain without being registered by the cerebral cortex.

Within the limbic system resides the regulatory mechanism of the innermost core of our being. Here is the seat of our sexuality, the impulse of attraction and aversion, our motivation and our moods, our memory, and creativity, as well as our autonomic nervous system.

Because the limbic system is directly connected to those parts of the brain that control heart rate, blood pressure, breathing, memory, stress levels, and hormone balance, essential oils can have some very profound physiological and psychological effects.

Also present in the limbic system of the brain is a gland called the amygdala. In 1989, it was discovered that the amygdala plays a major role in the storing and releasing of emotional trauma. The only way to stimulate this gland is with fragrance or the sense of smell. So now, with aromatherapy and essential oils, we are able to access the amygdala to release emotional trauma.

ESSENTIAL OIL CHEMISTRY

Chemistry? Are your eyes glazed over yet? It happens...yet if you're interested at all in the therapeutic use of essential oils, a little primer on your chemistry can be very useful. Not only will you better understand how and why essential oils work, but the great importance of using natural, high-quality oils - oils that are pure, properly distilled, and smell nice - will be made clear. It's not just an aromatherapy sales pitch; essential oils with exceptional bouquets have different chemical make-ups than flat or otherwise uninteresting oils. The differences can significantly affect the healing potency of therapeutic applications for you, your family and your loved ones. Much of the time, you can discern the difference of therapeutic value between two oils just by their aroma - one needn't always have the proof of fancy, expensive machines to make an educated choice.

So, why are essential oils called 'oils' anyway? They don't feel greasy, and they tend to evaporate completely, unlike common 'fixed' oils (such as olive, grape seed, hazelnut and the like). Essential oils and fixed oils share a similar chemical foundation: their structures are based on the linking of carbon and hydrogen atoms in various configurations. But this is really where the similarity ends. Fixed oils are made up of molecules comprised of three long chains of carbon atoms bound together at one end, called a triglyceride. Every fixed oil is made up of just a few different triglyceride arrangements - olive oil, for example, is primarily made up of oleic, linoleic and linolenic acids (the names of particular carbon-hydrogen chains forming the triglycerides). Their long-chain shape holds them in a liquid state which does not easily evaporate.

Essential oils are 'volatile' oils - oils that do easily evaporate. Their chains of carbon atoms to which the hydrogen atoms attach are not as long or heavy and are much more complex. Many essential oil structures are not really chains, but the ring, or multi-ringed shapes with diverse sub-units - called 'functional groups' - sticking out in various directions. Like their fixed oil counterparts, essential oils are lipophilic - meaning 'fat liking'. The fat-liking nature of both fixed and essential oils makes them easily absorbed by our bodies. Because of their typically smaller structures, however, essential oils are absorbed more rapidly than fixed oils, and can easily penetrate deep into the body. Despite their plant origins, this lipophilic nature of essential oils makes their profound healing action on the human body possible.

Most of the therapeutic activity of an essential oil can be attributed to the functional groups of the individual chemicals that make up the oil. There can be over a hundred identifiable molecules in one essential oil. Each of these molecules, as mentioned earlier, is a chain or ring (or multiple-ring) structure of carbon atoms linked together with hydrogen atoms bonded to them in various configurations.

Every chain or ring has a functional group attached to "a single atom or group of atoms that...has a profound influence on the properties of the molecule as a whole. It is often referred to as the chemically active center of the molecule".

As you can see, essential oils are really very complex in their chemical nature. There are nearly infinite possibilities of functional group and ring or chain combinations. One essential oil alone can be made up of hundreds of these different molecular arrangements. Don't worry, though! While it sounds complex, one needn't know all the precise chemical details to use essential oils therapeutically. When selecting between varieties of an essential oil, it is helpful to know that any particular oil is often composed of one or more primary molecular forms, with many minor or 'trace' constituents, and that all these molecules contribute to the oil's aroma and therapeutic action.

Many factors in an essential oil's production affect the total number and relative amounts of individual chemicals found in the final product. These include where the plant was grown, soil and climate conditions, time of harvest and distillation equipment, in addition to the time, temperature and pressure of distillation. This can give you an idea as to why two varieties of the same oil can smell so different: The full, beautiful bouquet of a fine essential oil will contain a myriad of notes, telling you that all natural components are present and in balanced amounts. Poorly distilled oils may lose some of the secondary constituents during production, and adulterated or synthetic oils may not have some of the trace components at all, detectable by your nose as a flat or uninteresting aroma.

To best understand this, researchers examine lavender essential oil; more than fifty individual molecules have been identified in pure lavender essential oil. The aromatherapist must remember that all of these chemicals found in pure and natural lavender oil work together to produce a therapeutic effect.

For example, the linalool molecule is antiviral and antibacterial; the linalyl acetate is also emotionally calming; other major components including cineol, limonene, pinene and others, all noted for specific biologic and aromatic activity. It is the combined, balanced, synergistic action of these chemicals that make pure, high-quality lavender such a great healer. No one chemical can be singled out and used to give the same profound results as the complete pure essential oil.

So how is this synergy reflected in lavender's aroma? Each of these chemicals has a unique smell; some are sweet, some are camphorous, some citrusy and some herbaceous. It is all these chemicals together, a precise amount of each, that gives each lavender variety its distinct aroma. And your nose knows this! One can tell the difference between a well-made, complex lavender oil with many notes within the aroma, and one that is flat or plain, which may be chemically imbalanced or missing some trace constituents.

One can easily tell the difference, for example, between common Lavendula Officinalis, and the finer Lavendula Angustifolia, which contains a higher proportion of sweet-smelling linalyl acetate and less sharp-smelling camphor. Further, lower quality lavender plants may occasionally be sprayed with linalool before harvest to enhance the production of linalyl acetate by the flowers. While the end-product may smell sweeter, the process actually creates an imbalance in the overall healing synergy of the primary and trace molecules. All these oils will be labeled 'Lavender' on the store shelf, yet the finer, natural lavender will have a more beautiful, balanced aromatic bouquet, and is considered the most holistically healing variety by the world's leading aromatherapy practitioners.

This, of course, is not only true of lavender essential oil. All essential oils are subject to similar variations in production methods or the manipulation of their molecular make-ups through the addition of synthetic chemicals. For the most therapeutic benefit, it is always best to use true, carefully-made essential oils. To do this, find a source that is dedicated to supplying only the highest grades of oils. Examine their product's aromatic quality and business practices so you are comfortable with their dedication to your health, not just their bottom line. Listen to your intuition and your own nose; they won't lie to you! With experience, your ability to discern between subtly different grades of oils will become more astute.

With even more education and skill, you'll start to recognize individual chemicals within an oils aroma and make the best decisions as to which oils will have the most profound therapeutic effects for you, your family, or in your professional practice.

CHAPTER TWO

WHAT ARE ESSENTIAL OILS?

Essential oils are highly concentrated liquids extracted from plant material - bark, berries, flowers, leaves, roots, seeds, or twigs - that are produced in several different ways.

The most common is a steam distillation, in which pressurized steam is passed through plant material, causing oils to evaporate out. The resulting mixture of oil and steam is condensed back into a liquid, and the oil is skimmed off.

Plants that are too fragile for steam distillation, such as jasmine, orange blossom, and rose; they can have their oils extracted using solvents. Oils created by this process are called absolutes and are generally used in perfumes or diffusers because the solvent residue makes most of them unsuitable for topical use.

A third method is carbon dioxide extraction. While these oils are technically absolutes, the pressurized carbon dioxide used as a solvent leaves no harmful residue and also creates thicker oil with a more rounded aroma.

Cold-pressed essential oils are those that have been extracted from fruit rind by grinding and pressing it.

Most essential oils do not have an indefinite shelf life: citrus oils will lose their efficacy after about six months, while most floral oils will last a year or maybe two. A few - cedar wood, patchouli, sandalwood, and vetiver - become better with age. You can refrigerate oils that you do not use often. It is also a good idea to store them away from sunlight, in small bottles with less airspace.

KNOW WHAT YOU'RE GETTING

The method of production is just one factor affecting the quality and price of these botanical extracts. Others include the rarity of the plant, how and where it was grown, how many plants are needed to produce the oil and the quality standards of the manufacturer.

Genuine rose oil, for example, is extremely expensive. This is simply because it takes 200 pounds of roses (approximately 60,000 flowers) to make 1 ounce of rose oil. That equals 30 roses for a single drop! If you are paying less than $80 for a 5-milliliter bottle of rose oil, it is either synthetic or it has been diluted with a carrier oil such as jojoba. Purchasing diluted oil is perfectly acceptable as long as you know what you are getting. Reputable suppliers will be upfront about whether their products are sold already diluted. Less reputable suppliers may sell an adulterated blend (for example, a small amount of rose oil mixed with cheaper rose geranium oil) and claim it is 100 percent rose oil.

It's also important to know that different varieties of the same plant can have different uses. For example, high-altitude French lavender is most often used in skin care products, while Bulgarian or English lavender is used in bath products, diffusers, or as a sleep aid. The variety called spike lavender is higher in camphor, which brings respiratory benefits. Lavandin is a hybrid of English lavender and spike lavender, and "40/42" is a blend of several varieties that is stretched with synthetic lavender oil and used by many soap makers.

We strongly recommend purchasing essential oils only from reputable distributors that specialize in aromatherapy supplies. Unfortunately, there are companies out there that rely more on outlandish claims than on the quality of their products and others that sell synthetic fragrance under the guise of essential oil. Here are a few red flags to watch for when choosing a product.

GRADING GUILE

Although essential oils do have therapeutic value, there are no regulatory standards for their production and no official grades of oil are assigned or recognized by any organization. Manufacturers and distributors who claim their oils are "therapeutic grade" are using this as a marketing term only, and it is meaningless as an indicator of the oil's quality.

SYNTHETIC SUBSTITUTION

Although we use aromatherapy to mean the therapeutic use of essential oils, the word is not formally defined or regulated by the US government.

As a result, it is legal to sell products labeled "aromatherapy" that do not contain essential oils, but only synthetic fragrance.

The synthetic fragrance may be described on a label as "aroma oil," "aromatic oil," "fragrance oil," or "perfume oil." These are all blended synthetic aromas that are diluted with mineral oil, propylene glycol, or vegetable oil and may also contain phthalates and other potentially toxic ingredients. Synthetics are much cheaper than essential oils, and their scent is much stronger. When you walk past a candle store and can smell the candles from outside, that is synthetic fragrance. There are a number of plants that cannot be used to produce essential oils: some examples are gardenia, lilac, and lily of the valley. So-called essential oils marketed under these names are always synthetic.

NUTRIENT NONSENSE

Some distributors make the claim that their essential oils deliver nutrients to the body. This is one thing these oils simply cannot do. Robert Tisserand, one of the most respected aromatherapists says, "Essential oils do not contain nutrients. They contain no vitamins, minerals, proteins, amino acids, carbohydrates, or any other type of nutrient." Claims that these oils can cure disease - even cancer - are also unsubstantiated by science, and you should be wary of any distributors willing to make such claims about their products.

If you intend to use essential oils, it is vitally important to think of them as any other healing tool: get proper training in their use, thoroughly research contraindications and interactions. Like anything else that can be applied to the body, essential oils can potentially cause harm. Remember, "natural" does not automatically mean a product is gentle or safe. And they should never, ever be taken internally unless you are under the care of a certified medical aromatherapist. This is not a license issued in the United States.

There are oils that must not be used on a person with high blood pressure and oils that interact with certain medications. Cypress and rosemary can be dangerous if a woman is pregnant or nursing. And some essential oils, such as wintergreen, can even be lethal if ingested.

One of the most common and dangerous misconceptions is that essential oils can be used neat (undiluted and applied directly to the skin) in skin care. I cannot emphasize enough that this is strongly discouraged by leading aromatherapists and all reputable manufacturers and distributors. No essential oil should ever be applied neatly to skin - not tea tree, not lavender, not any other kind of essential oil.

When these oils are applied neat, some people will have an immediate or delayed reaction, which can range from burning, irritation, or swelling to very major and serious health consequences. Other people will be unaffected - at first. Since the oil seems safe, they continue to use it. Over time, this causes the skin to become sensitized to that essential oil and the plant it comes from, with a longer-term, cumulative effect. When that happens, not only will the client be unable to use that oil again, they may not be able to use other products or foods that are related to it.

Correct use of essential oils for topical application always requires dilution, usually a strength of 6-15 drops of essential oil per ounce of whatever product it is being added to.

Citrus oils are good examples of how a wonderful oil can be harmful if used incorrectly. These oils have antiseptic properties and blend well with other products, but many citrus oils cause photosensitivity, and users should avoid direct sunlight for 12-72 hours after exposure. In addition, because citrus essential oils are created with the cold-pressed method, there will be traces of pesticide in the oil unless you are careful to buy organic. Whether citrus oil is organic or not, it can be irritating to the skin. For this reason, it's best to add citrus oils only to products that will be washed off, such as cleansers, not to a moisturizer or any other product intended to remain on the skin.

With the right knowledge and precautions, you can safely use essential oils. Take classes, read books that discuss each oil and its properties, and spend time researching the benefits and contraindications of the plants involved. You will soon be enjoying the sweet smell of successful aromatherapy.

WHAT BENEFITS DO PURE ESSENTIAL OILS PROVIDE?

1. Essential Oils are regenerating and oxygenating. They are the immune defense

properties of plants and are so small in molecular size that they can quickly penetrate the tissues of the skin.

2. Essential oils are lipid soluble and are capable of penetrating cell walls, even if they have hardened because of an oxygen deficiency. In fact, essential oils can affect every cell of the body within 20 minutes and are then metabolized like other nutrients.

3. Essential oils contain oxygen molecules which help to transport nutrients to the starving human cells. Because a nutritional deficiency is an oxygen deficiency, disease begins when the cells lack oxygen for proper nutrient assimilation. By providing the needed oxygen, essential oils also work to stimulate the immune system.

4. Essential oils are very powerful antioxidants. Antioxidants create an unfriendly environment for free radicals. They prevent all mutations, work as free radical scavengers, prevent fungus, and prevent oxidation in the cells.

5. Essential oils are antibacterial, anti-cancerous, anti-fungal, anti-infectious, anti-microbial, antitumoral, anti-parasitic, anti-viral, and

antiseptic. Essential oils have been shown to destroy all tested bacteria and viruses while simultaneously restoring balance to the body.

6.   Essential oils may detoxify the cells and blood in the body.

7.   Essential oils containing sesquiterpenes have the ability to pass the blood-brain barrier, enabling them to be effective in the treatment of Alzheimer's disease, Lou Gehrig's disease, Parkinson's disease, and multiple sclerosis.

8.   Essential oils are aromatic. When diffused, they provide air purification by removing metallic particles and toxins from the air, increasing atmospheric oxygen, increasing ozone and negative ions in the area, which inhibits bacterial growth; destroying odors from mold, cigarettes, and animals.

9.   Essential oils help promote emotional, physical and spiritual healing.

10.   Essential oils have a bio-electrical frequency that is several times greater than the frequency of herbs, food, and even the human body. Clinical research has shown that essential oils can quickly

raise the frequency of the human body, restoring it to its normal healthy level.

WHAT ENABLES PURE ESSENTIAL OILS TO PROVIDE SUCH INCREDIBLE BENEFITS?

Essential oils are chemically very heterogenetic; meaning they are very diverse in their effects and can perform several different functions. Synthetic chemicals are completely opposite in that they basically only have one action.

This gives essential oils a paradoxical nature which can be difficult to understand. However, they can be compared to another paradoxical group - human beings.

For example, a man can play many roles such as father, husband, friend, co-worker, accountant, school teacher, scoutmaster, etc...and so it is with essential oils. Lavender, for example, can be used for burns, insect bites, headaches, PMS, insomnia, stress, and so forth.

In beginning your journey into the realm of aromatherapy and essential oils it is very important to use only the purest oils available. Anything less than pure, may not produce the desired results and can, in some cases, be extremely toxic.

CHAPTER THREE

WAYS OF PRODUCING ESSENTIAL OILS

The use of essential oils to improve your overall health is called aromatherapy. The contents of essential oils are known as hormones, antibiotics, thermions (unseen scents) and recycling cells (essential to the existence of a live plant). Due to these properties, the immunity of plants to various diseases is heightened. Disease-causing bacteria and viruses are eliminated. Essential oils which are normally made from plants contain certain qualities that can benefit our overall health. There are two ways in which essential oils work; psychologically - by way of the body's sense of smell on the central nervous system by vaporizers or smelling of the oils; and physically - through the skin by mixing the oils for massage, foot baths or steam inhalation.

Aromatherapy is unique in the way in which it connects our overall health with the natural wealth of the world around us. The pleasure in itself is therapy, but aromatherapy goes further, by transforming therapy into pleasure. Use caution when using essential oils. Use caution when applying concentrated essential oils. Carrier oils are used when thinning essential oils for massage. Try not to use essential oils on sensitive areas such as the eyes. The curing of some diseases with oils may work well but for others may not be suitable. Always research the essential oils that you wish to use before doing so. Essential oils should be stored in a cool dark place in an airtight container.

COMMENTS ON ESSENTIAL OILS

Essential oils are sorted by their degree of lightness and subdivided into oils of the top, average and base categories. Essential oils of the top evaporate rapidly due to their lightness and care should be taken when storing them. Base oils evaporate the least rapidly. The most balanced and steady mixes are aroma-therapeutic mixes containing oils of the top, average and base category. In this chapter, we will explain how to make your own essential oils for massage or other applications.

NATURAL VS SYNTHETIC AROMATHERAPY OILS

Natural aromatherapy essential oils represent a high concentration of vegetative extracts derived by evaporation or extraction from flowers, berries, seeds, roots, bark or dried citrus peels. How much an essential oil is sold for depends on the amount of raw material required to produce the oil. The amount differs from plant to plant.

For example, from the petals of thirty roses, it is possible to receive only one drop of rose oil. This causes the high price, though there are also cheaper oils. Man-made or synthetic oils are made by combining certain artificially flavored oils in laboratories.

In technical language, flavored oils are actually not oils and are more likely artificial chemical compounds. These products usually carry exotic names of flowers or fruit from which they have not been derived. True peach or strawberry oils do not exist. Even though their aroma is pleasant, flavored oils do not possess any healing qualities or any properties of plants. They cannot be used for medicinal reasons and some can be dangerous when applied to the skin. As a precaution, it is suggested that you not use these substances for aromatherapy applications as there is no information on their safety.

WAYS OF PRODUCING AROMATHERAPY OILS

The most common method of producing aromatherapy essential oils is steam distillation. One method of direct distillation is where the steam distillatory is loaded with raw vegetative material. Under high pressure, the steam is piped into the distillatory and the vegetative matter mixes with the steam. The steam and vegetative matter condense into a liquid on top of which floats the essential oils. The water is then removed leaving the essential oils. Cold Pressing is applied to raw materials to derive citric oils. This is basically a soft pressure method where the oils are pressed out of the citric peels. Carrier oils are produced in the same way by pressing seeds. Solvent extraction is the method of extraction using special solvents. The resulting absolute oils are extremely pure. It is a delicate procedure to remove an aromatic substance from vegetative matter with solvents. The wax-like residue that remains when the solvents are removed is mixed with alcohol and is carefully heated.

Following this is a filtration procedure in which the wax is removed. The pure oils remain once the alcohol is removed. Every absolute oil carries a quality certificate.

ESSENTIAL OILS VS ABSOLUTE OILS

Aromatherapy essential oils possess a high concentration of aromatic vegetative extracts. Steam distillation is the normal method by which essential oils are derived from vegetative matter. Citrus oils are produced by cold pressing the fruit peels. Absolute oils are obtained by a method of extraction using solvents at the end of which all-soluble material is removed and are usually more concentrated than essential oils.

INFUSED AROMATHERAPY ESSENTIAL OILS

Plant flowers are submerged in olive or soy oils for a reasonable period of time This allows the oils to receive the essence of the flower and use it for the manufacture of infused oils. For producing carrot oil, the extract of the root crop is soaked in soy oil for the most effective utilization of its aromatic properties.

CARRIER OILS

Carrier or base oils are vegetable based and are very high in quality and nutrition. When combined with essential oils they allow the pure oils to be used for massage and body and skin care. Carrier oils can be obtained by cold pressing seeds, nuts, barks, and grains.

PURE AROMATHERAPY ESSENTIAL OILS - 3% MIX

In their pure form, some essential oils are too concentrated to use so manufacturers dilute them. Generally, essential oil manufacturers make the essential oils useable by combining them with carrier oils in a 3% mix.

MASSAGE OIL BLENDS

Essential oils used for massage come ready to use as they are blended with carrier oils. These carrier oils are derived from almonds or grains, apricots, and seeds of fruits. These are added to the oil of young wheat which raises the stability of the mix and increases shelf life.

HERBAL CREAMS

Well-researched formulas of creams consist of essential oils and natural extracts from select vegetation. High-grade lanolin is used as a basis for many formulas.

ESSENTIAL OILS FOR BEGINNERS

For the beginner, the safe use and buying of essential oils is necessary. Essential oils are not only used for aromatherapy but also in the food and perfume industries and as such there are different qualities of oils. When buying essential oils to use in healing you should only buy 100% pure essential oils.

It is also recommended that pregnant woman do not use essential oils, and those that suffer from epilepsy should be careful with which oils they use. Although with care and understanding most essential oils are safe to use, the list below will detail those that are the best essential oils for beginners.

1. Lavender essential oil: Botanical name Lavendula Angustifolia; probably the most widely known and can be used for so many ailments. Lavender can be used as an analgesic, an antidepressant, an antiviral, an antispasmodic, a deodorant, a sedative, a diuretic, and can also be used for arthritis, rheumatism, and decongestant; to name just a few.

Lavender is well known for its sedative properties and helps in the treatment of conditions such as depression, insomnia, hysteria, and stress. It is also helpful in treating headaches and migraines, for coughs and colds, treating bites and small wounds and is undoubtedly a very necessary item for the treatment of superficial burns and sunburn.

Because of its low toxicity lavender is considered one of the best essential oils to use safely on children. Lavender can also be used for skin conditions such as dermatitis, eczema, and acne.

2. Chamomile, German: Botanical name, Matricaria recutita. There are 2 types of Chamomile used in Aromatherapy, German and Roman, I am giving the German here as it is non-toxic, non-irritant, non-sensitizing and safe to use on children. Chamomiles properties include use as an anti-allergenic, anti-inflammatory, antispasmodic and a sedative.

German Chamomile can be used to help treat inflammation, infected cuts, muscular pain, arthritis, and sprains. It can also be used to help treat many skin problems such as eczema, psoriasis and any other itchy dry skin problems.

German Chamomile is most commonly used with a carrier oil in massage, but can also be used in hot and cold compresses.

3. Eucalyptus: The properties of Eucalyptus include analgesic, anti-bacterial, anti-inflammatory, antiseptic, decongestant and antiviral. Eucalyptus can be used to help with concentration but is mainly used for its antiviral properties in treating asthma, bronchitis, coughs, and colds, and clearing the airways and loosening phlegm. Eucalyptus is non-toxic and a non-irritant.

Another good use of eucalyptus is to add a few drops of the oil to a spray bottle of water and use it around the house as a room spray and also on your kitchen benches. It can also be used when washing your pet's bedding.

4. Tea Tree: Botanical name Melaleuca alternifolia. Tea Tree oils properties include use as an antiseptic, fungicidal, antimicrobial and stimulant. Tea tree oil is non-toxic, non-irritant but may cause sensitivity in some individuals.

Tea tree oil along with lavender would be a great addition to your first aid kit.

The oil aids in combating infectious organisms such as bacteria, viruses, and fungi. It can be used to clean dirty wounds so they don't become infected, used in a glass of water and gargled for throat infections, mouth ulcers and to help eliminate bad breath, and can be used for athlete's foot and thrush. It can also be used with lavender in the treatment of acne and is used on the hair to help control dandruff and head lice.

Use a cotton bud with 1 drop of tea tree oil to dab on stings and bites.

5. Rosemary: Rosemary is generally non-toxic, non-irritant and non-sensitizing but it needs to be used with caution as it may not be suitable for people with epilepsy or high blood pressure and pregnant women should not use it.

Rosemary's properties include use as an antidepressant, astringent, diuretic, stimulant and tonic.

Rosemary is considered one of the best tonics for the nervous system and it also helps with memory. It can be used in a bath or massage to relieve muscular aches and pains, rheumatism and arthritis. Rosemary can also be used in shampoos and conditioners as it helps hair growth.

This list of best essential oils is by no means exhaustive. There are many other essential oils available, but for the beginner, these are recommended because they are non-toxic, non-irritating and non-sensitizing and they have many uses, on their own or blended.

ESSENTIAL OIL SAFETY TIPS

Aromatherapy is one of the safest therapies if used under the directions of a qualified Physician. Special attention should be paid while applying essential oil. Some essential oils should be avoided at certain times and others should be handled with care. Here a few safety tips for the use of aromatherapy oils.

1. Always thoroughly research the essential oil or oils you are working with. Some essential oils should not be taken internally, while others should never be put on the skin "neat" (i.e., undiluted). Some essential oils could have a negative effect on those with high blood pressure, epilepsy, and other medical conditions. There are also essential oils that should only be used for a short period of time, and others should not be used in a diffuser and/or nebulizer.

2. Keep essential oils away from children and pets. Treat the essential oils as if they were prescription medicines -- helpful in the right circumstances, but potentially harmful to others.

3. Do not put essential oils on your skin and go into sunlight unless you are certain it is safe to do so. Some essential oils, such as bergamot (citris bergamia), Angelica (Angelica Archangelica), lemon (Citrus limon), tangerine (Citrus reticulata) and others may cause a rash or dark pigmentation after

sun exposure. Avoid tanning booths as well when using these photo-sensitive essential oils.

4. Essential oils can interact with prescription medications. If you are on any prescription medication, you must research the potential interactions of your medication(s) and the essential oil(s) you choose to use. Remember that you do not have to take an essential oil internally for it to have effects on your whole body. Essential oils applied externally may also affect your entire body.

5. If you are pregnant, consult with a qualified aromatherapist and/or medical professional before using any essential oils.

6. Never put an essential oil undiluted on your skin unless you are absolutely certain that it is safe to do so. For example, lavender (Lavandula augustifolia) essential oil and tea tree (Melaleuca alternifolia) essential oil is generally considered to be safe to apply neat to the skin, but many others are not safe to use this way. And remember that "skin" is not the same thing as "mucosal skin". Mucosal skin is the skin inside your mouth, nose, vagina, and rectum. Mucosal skin is usually too sensitive for

neat/undiluted application of even the safest essential oils.

7. Before putting an essential oil, neat or diluted, on a large area of your skin, put a tiny amount on a sensitive area, such as your inner arm, as a test. Wait 30 minutes or more to ensure there is no burning or irritation. Some aromatherapy professionals advocate waiting 24 hours before trying the oil on a larger area of skin. This is often referred to as a "skin patch test".

8. Never put essential oil anywhere near your eyes! It will burn horribly and could damage the sensitive eye surfaces. Avoid touching your eyes until you have washed your hands following essential oil handling.

9. Avoid putting undiluted essential oils near your lips, as it will burn terribly. If you are taking essential oils internally, place them in an empty vegetable or gelatin capsule with an eye dropper.

Remember to read about any essential oil before taking it internally. It is always better to err on the side of caution and not take an oil internally if you are not 100% certain the essential oil is safe to ingest.

10. Never put essential oils, in any form, in the ear canal except under the supervision of a qualified medical professional.

11. Wear gloves when handling undiluted essential oils. The oil will create holes in latex gloves, so it's best to wear vinyl gloves.

12. Wash your hands thoroughly with soap and water after handling essential oils.

13. If your skin burns from the application of a neat or diluted essential oil, **do not wash the area with water!** Water will simply spread the oil over a larger area of skin. Use a carrier oil, such as olive oil or jojoba oil to dilute the essential oil. Gently rub some carrier oil into the irritated skin. The burning sensation should calm down within a few minutes.

14. Never leave a candle diffuser unattended, and do not let nebulizing diffusers run for long periods of time by themselves.

15. Do not add essential oils to candle wax unless you are 100% certain it is safe. Some essential oils have very low flash-points and are not safe to use around a flame.

16. Keep essential oils away from any open flame or potential spark.

17. Keep your bottles of essential oil in tightly closed, dark-colored containers, stored in a cool, dark, dry place. Do not expose them to sunlight.

18. Do not add undiluted essential oils to bath water. The undiluted oil will float on top of the water and can irritate sensitive skin.

This list of safe aromatherapy essential oil safety tips is not meant to be exhaustive. Consultation with a qualified aromatherapist and/or medical practitioner before using any essential oil is advisable.

HOW TO USE ESSENTIAL OILS?

You can use them directly on the skin but take care of your children and dilute with some natural oils before applying directly to their skin. However, most of them are considered harmless for topical application and they tend to reduce skin irritations due to their anti-inflammatory properties. Some of them are the oil of clove, rose oils, eucalyptus and Thyme. For topical applications, if you deem necessary, you can also fit a roller to the bottle and use it on your skin.

You can also inhale their aroma either directly from the bottle or with the help of an inhaler to enjoy its soothing benefits.

It is quite difficult to encompass all the benefits of using essential oils in a single chapter because they are nearly countless. However, some of the most common ones have been discussed briefly below:

1. For home cleaning and other related purposes

The oils like cinnamon, citronella, eucalyptus, tea tree oils, clove, rosemary and others find application for home purification and cleaning purposes. While the eucalyptus and citronella are extensively used as mosquito repellents, others like clove and rosemary are mainly used to purify the air in your homes and provide an excellent aromatic atmosphere to enhance your senses. Lemon oil and tea tree oil mixed with water are mainly used for cleaning and disinfecting. You can also use cinnamon oil as a natural disinfectant.

2. For use at Spas

Yes, lavender, the name you hear often is nothing but an essential oil used in spa therapy for their exceptional relaxation properties. They are said to improve sleep, thus getting rid of that awful nightmare. Lavender is also a natural stress reliever. For maximum effects, rub a small quantity of oil on the palm of your hands and breathe in the odor. You are bound to feel relaxed and considerably relieved of stress after some time. Cedarwood, along with lavender are also used in body massage treatments while eucalyptus oil finds application in foot massages. You can also improve your yoga sessions by inhaling the beautiful aroma of sandalwood oil a few minutes before you step into the class.

3. For beauty and skin care

Tree tea oil mixed with some amount of honey can help reduce acne. A drop of peppermint oil helps reduce problems of bad breath. Add cedarwood, lavender oil or Basil to your shampoo in order to get rid of an itchy scalp. Oils from the lemon can be used as a natural teeth whitening element. You can also use grapefruit and lavender oil in your facial scrub.

4. Therapeutic benefits

Essential oils are said to have natural healing power. In the remote past, when people did not have medicines or even the herbal treatment, they used essential oils to cure ailments. Even today, they act as a relief to migraine headaches, bronchitis, asthma problems and reduce motion sickness.

CHAPTER FOUR

WHERE TO BUY ESSENTIAL OILS

There are various places that you can get essential oils. If you are a health or organic food shopper then you have probably seen essential oils for sale at health food stores or with the vitamins and supplements at a regular grocery store. However, if you are like most people you probably didn't know that they were there or if you did, you didn't know how to use them or how the essential oils that you find at the store are different from other brands.

It can be very confusing to know where the best places are to buy essential oils. There are lots of brands and many of them say 100% pure on them. However, there is no regulation of these products in the United States and so even though it may say 100% pure, it does not necessarily mean that they are. It is possible for there to be additives, filers, and other chemicals from pesticides still in them.

So how do you determine the best place to buy them?

Personally, I have a brand that I really prefer but there are other brands that can work quite well too. Here are a few things to think about when buying essential oils.

1. What is the smell? This is the first clue to a quality product. All you need to do is take off the lid and smell it. Do you smell weeds, grass, or anything other than pure oil? This smell is pretty obvious, especially with the more common oils. For example, most people have a pretty good sense of what lemon, lavender or peppermint smell like.

2. What does it say on the bottle? Does it say 100% pure? If not, then for sure it is not the best. Does it list ingredients? If so, does it say that there is anything other than oil in the bottle? Does it say for external use only? If so, this may be a clue that the oil is not really 100% pure. Not all oils can be ingested even if they are pure; however, common oils such as lemon, lavender, and peppermint should be able to be ingested if they are 100% pure.

3. What is the price? Many people have a tendency to buy things based only on price. I am no different. I love a good bargain just as much as the next person. However, I have learned that sometimes a

higher price is worth it. This is especially true with essential oils. If the price seems really cheap then more than likely you are not getting the best product.

The best places to buy essential oils vary according to your intended purpose. If you are looking for a perfume quality oil then you can buy them at the grocery store. If you are looking for a message type oil then there are spas that offer them for sale. Or if you need them for health and wellness then you can try the ones at a health food store.

HOW TO STORE YOUR ESSENTIAL OILS

Many people enjoy creating their own natural health and beauty products, ranging from face creams and body butters right through to homemade treatments for various conditions. Some of the most vital products for this creation of these homemade items are extracts and essential oils, which often provide a number of benefits.

When it comes to storing these items at home, however, it is essential to abide by a few rules to ensure that they last as long as possible. This is because many essential oils and other natural products such as almond or argan oil need to be kept in certain conditions to ensure their longevity.

The first thing to remember when storing your natural products is that they should absolutely be kept out of direct sunlight. This is for a number of reasons, the first being that sunlight can actually cause light damage to the products in question, which can mean that its beneficial qualities are diminished or even entirely destroyed.

Many essential oils and plant extracts are quite costly to buy, therefore it is certainly important to preserve your investment by storing them so they last as long as possible. Keeping products out of direct sunlight is certainly the first step in doing this.

For this reason, many suppliers of these types of products will package their essential oils in dark-colored glass bottles, particularly amber colored or deep cobalt blue colored bottles. These will help limit the impact of the sun's rays on an oil, but they cannot provide complete protection, so again, it is essential (pun intended) to avoid sunlight altogether if possible.

It is also important to note that many oils are very acidic and therefore can eat through plastic bottles.

This is not always the case, as some products such as almond or argan oil are perfectly safe when stored in plastic, but citrus oils are best stored in glass.

For this reason, when you buy a product, ask the vendor what type of container it comes in, as this will help you decide if it needs to be repackaged for storage purposes. The retailer will often be able to provide you with advice on whether certain products can be stored in plastic or not, or if the glass is preferable.

Another way that sunlight can damage oils is by heating them up, as these products are usually quite unstable and need to be kept at a low and steady temperature in order for them to conserve all their beneficial properties.

It is not only sunlight which can cause this issue, as heat from radiators or open fires can also have a negative effect. Similarly, temperature fluctuations are not very good for your natural oils and extracts, so try to keep them in a cool place where the temperature does not fluctuate significantly.

Many experts often recommend that essential oils and certain other extracts are kept in a refrigerator for best results. This will stop heat damage and ensure that all the beneficial properties of an oil are retained as long as possible.

However, this is not always possible for everyone, in which case it is a wise idea to invest in a little storage box or tray where all your natural products can be kept, placing it in a cool, dark place. Whether you have argan oil to store or lavender essential oil, following these techniques will ensure that your products last as long as possible.

If you have any doubts about how to store your raw extracts or any of the natural beauty products that you create, it is strongly recommended to talk to a trusted retailer of natural extracts. He or she will be able to guide you in selecting the right storage containers and the best storage conditions for any given item.

CHAPTER FIVE

POPULAR OILS WITH HEALING PROPERTIES

Aromatherapy uses essential oils for treating common diseases. This chapter discusses some popular essential oils with healing properties.

1. Juniper

Juniper oil has been used for hundreds of years as a household disinfectant.

Juniper essential oil is helpful for:

a. Acne: Mix four drops of juniper oil with 2 tsp (10 ml) of carrier oil and gently massage the face and neck (and shoulders if acne is present there).

b. Cystitis and Period Pain: Blend into a carrier oil and rub the lower abdomen at regular intervals. Also, add five or six drops of your bathwater and soak for at least fifteen minutes.

c. Muscular/rheumatic pain: Use for massage or in the bath

d. Poor blood circulation: Juniper is stimulating oil. Use in the bath, or in a carrier oil, daily to improve circulation.

e. Stress and anxiety: Use for massage, in the bath or in a vaporizer.

2. Jasmine

This essential oil is extracted from the flower of the jasmine bush. This oil has a beautiful, exotic aroma and is really helpful in cases of extreme nervous anxiety and stress. It is one of the most expensive oils and is often used in the manufacture of perfumes.

Jasmine essential oil is helpful for:

a. Dry, sensitive, mature skin: Use in a carrier oil for massage or add a couple of drops to rosewater and use as a freshener.

b. Nervous exhaustion: Use in a carrier oil for massage or inhale.

c. Period pain: Use in a carrier oil and massage the lower abdomen and back at regular intervals.

3. Lemon

It takes 3000 lemons to produce 2 pounds (1 kg) of essential oil. It is extracted by pressing the rind of the fruit.

Lemon essential oil is helpful for:

a. Bites and stings: Dab neat oil onto the bite or sting.

b. Catarrh/colds: Mix in a carrier oil and massage the face and head, or inhale.

c. Chilblains: Mix into a carrier oil and gently rub the affected areas three to four times a day. Or use in a footbath, soaking the feet for fifteen minutes.

d. Cold sores: Dab with a cotton bud which has been soaked in 2 tsp (10 ml) of boiled water to which 5 drops of oil have been added.

e. Mouth ulcers: Dab on the neat oil, or make a gargle adding five drops to a medium size glass of water.

f. Warts: Dab with a cotton bud soaked in neat essential oil several times a day.

Essential oils are aromatic oils extracted from plants and have many therapeutic benefits. Essential oils are used to soothe the skin, heal cuts, eliminate pimples, and help you relax, relieve digestive problems and even cure colds and flu.

For therapeutic purposes, only the purest oils will do. Unfortunately, there are many companies out there selling low-quality oils and you should only buy from a source that you trust. Like with anything else, you get what you get what you pay for so if an oil seems to be priced quite cheaply, it's probably not a good quality oil for medicinal purposes.

When using essential oils, it's important to remember that these oils are strong and should not be applied directly to the skin. Mix them with base oils like almond or wheat germ oil to reduce their potency.

ESSENTIAL OILS FOR HEALING AND THERAPY

1. Lavender

Perhaps the most popular of the essential oils, lavender has many uses. It is a great topical treatment which can help heal cuts, bruises, and burns and is also a wonderful aid to help you relax and can be a natural sleep inducer.

2. Peppermint

Peppermint oil is great for treating digestive complaints and may be used in preparations for freshening breath.

3. Tea Tree and Eucalyptus

These oils have long been used to treat a variety of respiratory ailments. They can be massaged into the chest or used in an oil burner and help relieve congestion making them excellent oils to use for colds. Tea tree oil is also a natural antiseptic and can be dabbed on cuts, bites, and stings. It can be used to treat spots and pimples and can be used to gargle but should never be swallowed.

4. Geranium

Geranium oil has been used for years as a pain reliever.

5. Rosemary and Thyme

Not only do these herbs taste good but they have wonderful antiseptic properties and can be good for healing problems with the skin.

6. Citronella

Citronella oil is a natural insect repellent so it's no wonder they use it in the manufacture of oils and sprays as well as candles to repel insects.

To protect your pet against fleas, try soaking his or her collar in citronella oil. To help keep down insects in summer, buy some citronella Geraniums and put them on your porch or deck.

7. Garlic

Garlic is another natural insect repellent and is vital in helping to keep your immune system healthy. It can be a great way to help prevent colds and viruses naturally. It also has antibacterial and antifungal properties. And it tastes good too!

8. Patchouli

This fragrant oil smells great when used in an oil burner but it is also a great topical treatment for eczema and dandruff.

9. Ylang-ylang

This is another fragrant oil that can be burned for its aroma and is also reputed to relieve stress, palpitations, and high blood pressure.

10. Orange Oil

Used as an aromatherapy, it is reputed to help with depression and nervous tension.

11. Cinnamon

This tasty herb is becoming popular for many treatments, but it's great when used for aromatherapy. Mix it with orange oil and you'll have a wonderful homey smell in your house. As a topical oil, it is excellent for warts and viral infections.

If you are really ambitious, you can grow these herbs yourself and collect the oil by stewing large amounts in pure water. Collect the steam and let it cool. The essential oils will rise to the top of the drained water and can be collected with an eyedropper.

CHAPTER SIX

AROMATHERAPY FOR PETS

Pets can enjoy the therapeutic effects of aromatherapy as much as humans can. Aside from possibly eliminating bad odors and giving your pet a pleasant perfume, essential oils also serve many practical functions such as boosting your pet's immune system, fighting off bacteria and viruses, preventing the growth of yeasts and molds and repelling insects.

Aromatherapy is used by enthusiasts, groomers and pet salons to treat mild ailments such as skin inflammations, itchy skin, ear infections, rashes, bad breath, flatulence and motions sickness. Psychologically, certain oils also have a calming or relaxing effect on animals. For example, lavender oil not only helps cats repel insects but it also makes them feel sleepy or content. Roman chamomile can be used to treat an ear infection as well as soothe the nerves of a dog in pain.

Essential oils are also frequently used as home remedies. However, before you attempt to use aromatherapy on your own pets, keep in mind that essential oils are always diluted before they are applied to a pet's skin or sprayed on their coat. Almond oil, olive oil, and jojoba oil are common base oils to which a few drops of the essential oil is added. Usually, all that is needed is about one ounce of the base oil combined with two to three drops of the essential oil.

Essential oils can also be diluted in a spray bottle and misted onto the pet or the pet's bedding. You can simply dilute a few drops in distilled water or you can use water and a mixture of aloe, witch hazel or cider vinegar. The traditional recommendation is to use 20 to 30 drops of oil per eight ounces of liquid. Any less might not be effective and any more might be toxic to the pet.

Oils can also be diluted in vodka or brandy and dabbed on the bottom of the pet's paws or on an acupressure point such as the tips of the ears. This is the technique to use if you are dealing with a panicky pet. Never feed your pet alcohol or essential oil directly.

Essential oils are also effective flea and tick repellents and are nearly as effective as sprays and powders that contain a lot of toxic chemicals. Oils such as peppermint, citronella, lavender, eucalyptus, lemon, geranium, bay and myrrh have been components of herbal flea sprays and flea collars for many years. You can easily make your own flea and tick spray by combining about 25 drops of any of these oils into eight ounces of water. Shake the mixture well and spray it on your pet, being careful to shield its eyes from the mist. This mixture can also be sprayed anywhere that you suspect there may be a breeding bug infestation.

When using essential oils it is also important for you to remember that a dog or cat's sense of smell is much more acute than our own. Signs that an aromatherapy treatment is too overwhelming for your pet are tearing eyes, sneezing, pacing or whining. Cats may lick themselves excessively and dogs may rub their head on the ground in order to escape the smell. Many pets also have allergies to essential oils.

For instance, chamomile is related to the ragweed plant, which is a common allergen for both pets and humans. This is why it is so important to use a mild solution at first and use your powers of observation the first few times you use an essential oil mixture on a pet.

Essential oils for pets is the all-natural healthy approach to help improve the quality of life for your dog using aromatherapy. How can you be sure aromatherapy works? Bake some homemade cookies and see if it puts you in a better mood! Now imagine you could smell as well as your dog. Essential oils for pets take the essential oils from plants which is the 100% oil that a plant naturally produces and used in various ways to improve naturally the emotional or physical well-being of your beloved dog. There are many different oils that can be used for different purposes on your dog.

To mention just a few;

1. Eucalyptus oil helps with soothing respiratory ailments.

2. Frankincense helps to boost the immune system and it helps with tumors and warts.

3. Lavender is used in treating cuts and burns. Inhaling lavender can help in calming an overactive puppy.

4. Oregano is strong antibacterial oil that is effective when it is inhaled.

5. Lemon oil can be used as an alternative to citronella oil. It acts as an insect repellant.

6. Naioli is used as an alternative to tea tree oil. Its topical application helps in skin allergies and helps in healing ear infections.

7. Rosemary is used for arthritis, in repelling fleas and lice. It is also used in skin irritation.

8 Peppermint oil can be used to make a sluggish lazy dog more active and lose weight.

These are just a few of the essential oils that can be used in various mixtures to improve the quality of your pet's health in natural ways. A detailed guide to using and mixing the oils is always recommended so that you do not harm your dog in any way.

NOTE: Animals are more sensitive to essential oils, and while in most cases it won't harm them if applied without dilution, it may cause discomfort or skin sensitivity particular with some of the "hotter" oils. For horses and dogs, dilute the oils mentioned above with one part essential oil to one part carrier oil. For cats, you should dilute the above oils one part essential oil to 10 parts carrier oil. Olive or coconut oil make great carrier oils for animals.

CHAPTER SEVEN

ESSENTIAL OILS FOR CHILDREN

Generally speaking, essential oils are known to be safe for use if it has the right solution. However, they can be very strong to the skin because their concentration is very high. Therefore, you should be very cautious before using them, especially for your baby's delicate skin. First consult a trusted aromatherapist and strictly follow the safety guidelines before applying any kind of essential oil to your child, because their skin is very sensitive and susceptible to harsh components. Likewise, be very careful when choosing carrier oils or base oils. Choose only the gentle ones.

A lot of essential oils that are being used these days have only a mild level of toxicity and are considered safe for adults. However, they still may not be safe for your children because their immune system is still young and not yet fully developed. Therefore, you should make sure that you are using the safe ones. Babies and small young children have a huge possibility of being allergic to different kinds of foods.

Some volatile oils are also likely to cause unpleasant effects. This is why parents should be extra careful when choosing essential oils in aromatherapy for their children. Some of the safer essential oils are tea tree and lavender, but you will still need some intensive care before using them. If you notice that your child feels uncomfortable or irritated with the smell of a certain volatile oil, stop using that oil at once and do not use it again because your baby might be allergic to it. If your child does not like the smell of a certain essential oil, it also has a great potential to be not the right oil for him or her. Therefore, parents should find time to try searching for a safer alternative for that essential oil.

If you are using aromatherapy while your baby is still breast feeding, make sure that you do not apply any amount of essential oil on or near your nipples. If you do, your baby will have a large tendency to ingest it and can cause them harm.

There are certain volatile oils that should not be applied or used even with a diffuser on children who are sick or recently had an illness, because some of them are very strong oils and are known to be extremely dangerous for both adults and children. There are certain oils that should never be used in aromatherapy.

It is therefore very important to check the warnings and precautions on the labels before using them.

Oils can really benefit children. Keep them happy by employing these essential oils:

1. German Chamomile: Put a few drops in your child's bath at night to calm them down. German Chamomile oil promotes rest. Start off with a small amount of the bath because too much oil can irritate your child's skin.

2. Peppermint: This oil promotes good digestion. It can also be handy for children with headaches. Peppermint is meant to only be used on children older than 30 months.

3. Lavender: This is a favorite essential. Parents enjoy the oil's healing properties, and children enjoy the fabulous smell. Lavender can be used for the cuts, stings, and scrapes that children often get when playing outside.

4. Eucalyptus: Colds happen all during the year. They can still happen during the summer, much to our dismay. Eucalyptus oil does wonders as a decongestant and immune stimulant.

5. Lemon: This citrus oil works great in a room diffuser. It can help bodies fight off infections. The smell is delicious and doubles as an air freshener. Never apply this oil to your skin directly as it can irritate it.

6. Melaleuca oil: Melaleuca oil is an all-purpose natural essential oil. Melaleuca oil is the best choice for a first aid kit. It works great for cuts and scrapes, reducing pain, healing and disinfecting. Melaleuca oil can even be used to clean your home if you want. It may be a good idea for children with chores they need to do around the home.

ESSENTIAL OIL SAFETY

Essential oils are highly concentrated substances that come to us from the plant world; specifically from the leaves, flowers, roots, and fruits of aromatic plants as discussed earlier.

Here are essential oil usage safety tips:

1. Dilute before using

Always dilute essential oils before applying to the skin, as applying them 'neat', (in their pure form), can cause skin irritation, rashes, and allergic reactions. Lavender and tea tree oils are often cited as being exceptions to this rule, but in most situations, diluting these oils is still the preferred method. A general rule of thumb is to add one drop of essential oil per teaspoon of high quality, cold pressed vegetable oil, such as sweet almond or grapeseed oil. If you want to create an aromatherapy bath, add two to four drops to a warm (not hot) bath. If blending several oils together, treat the blend as a single oil; in other words, use no more than four drops of the blend in a bath, or one drop of the blend to a teaspoon of vegetable oil.

2. Patch test

When trying out a new aromatherapy oil, it's a good idea to do a patch test first, especially if you have sensitive skin or allergies. Mix one drop of the oil you're testing into a teaspoon of base oil and dab a tiny amount on the inside of the arm or wrist area. Wait 24 hours to ensure no redness or irritation occurs.

3. Quality matters

It's important to buy high-quality oils, and not confuse essential oils with fragrance oils, which are synthetic, not natural products. Some products sold as pure oils are diluted in cheaper carrier oils or are adulterated in some other way. Again, read product labels carefully but be aware that labels may not disclose full information. Become familiar with the botanical names of the oils you want to use and never purchase an oil that is not labeled with the botanical name, as well as the common name.

Some Cautions:

- If you are pregnant or nursing, consult with your doctor before using aromatherapy.
- Keep aromatherapy products out of reach of children and pets.
- Keep essential oils away from your eyes and mucous membranes.
- Be careful around furniture, as undiluted oils can damage varnished surfaces.
- Citrus oils, such as lemon, tangerine, orange, bergamot, and grapefruit are photosensitizing - which means they can induce sunburn. Do not use

these oils before exposure to sunlight or tanning beds.

- Do not use essential oils internally, unless under the supervision of a doctor or qualified practitioner. Remember that these oils are concentrated substances, and could be dangerous if ingested. Using the oils in massage or inhalation is safer and very effective.

Hopefully, this list of cautions won't put you off from experimenting with aromatherapy. Essential oils are versatile, powerful, emotionally and physically balancing, and of course, they smell fabulous. Enjoy experimenting with them safely.

ESSENTIAL OILS CHILDREN SHOULD AVOID

Volatile oil that should never be used anytime by adults and children alike are the essential oils from the following:

- Acorus calamus
- American wormseed and mugwort
- Amygdalus communis amara or bitter almond
- Anise
- Bay laurel

- Birch
- Basil
- Black pepper
- Bay
- Cedarwood
- Clary sage
- Clove
- Citronella
- Dwarf juniper
- Horseradish root
- Lovage
- Marjoram
- Myrrh
- Nutmeg
- Oregano
- Ruta graveolens or rue
- Sassafras oil
- Scented fern
- Sweet fennel
- Sage
- Thyme
- Wormwood

CHAPTER EIGHT

ESSENTIAL OIL DILUTION

There is no better thing than essential oils that can be put to use in multiple ways. Anyone can use essential oil according to his or her needs. A variety of essential oils are available in the market to satisfy the diverse, never-ending needs of people.

Different people use different essential oils as per their need. The sensitivity of skin varies from person to person. You need to stay aware of the fact that essential oils may harm your body if your skin is sensitive. But, no need to fear. Now, you can use essential oil dilution to dilute the concentration of essential oil in case you have sensitive skin.

Essential oil is made from all natural ingredients so that there are no side effects. Essential oils are quite easy to use and have many benefits attached to them. They are commonly used for easy inhalation, includings steam inhalation that can help with cold and influenza, massage that help in toning the body, room freshening, baths and many more.

It is true that pure essential oils are volatile oils and can easily penetrate the skin. Using essential oil may cause skin irritation or sensitivity if not properly diluted in a carrier oil or if used in high concentrations. Children and the elderly are especially sensitive and are specifically found to be sensitive to neat essential oil.

Essential oil dilution acts as a mode to diminish the strength of the essential. People who experience skin sensitivity to even mild essentials oils can choose appropriate essential oil dilution. Whenever you use an essential oil for the first time, make sure to test yourself for sensitivity by applying your chosen essential oils in a dilution only to a small skin area before using on a larger area of the body.

With regards to stkin sensitivity, the type of essential oil used and the degree of results you desire determines the dilution needed in the essential oil. Make sure to take a careful, measured approach when using any essential oil and adjust both the quantity of oilst used and the amount of dilution in accordance with the body's response that will help you make the best use of the benefits of the essential oil.

Use of essential oil dilution does not affect the benefits of essential oil in any manner. It is just a means to make essential oils suitable for all, even for people with sensitive skin. It is always recommended to buy the essential oil from a trusted source, which serves only pure essential oils to derive essential oil benefits in the best possible manner.

CONCLUSION

Aromatherapy is the most ancient way of holistic healing. Aromatherapy is closely related to essential oils. Pure essential oils are highly concentrated essences of plants. The use of pure essential oils assists in health and wellbeing by comforting the mind, relieving stress, balance emotions and provide support for numerous physical ailments. Pure essential oils are the right ingredient for maintaining a healthy mind, body, and spirit.

Pure essential oils work on our emsotional states through the olfactory system. When pure essential oils are inhaled, they are immediately transferred to the emotional center of our brain. Pure essential oils are also used in massages. Here they are not inhaled but absorbed by the skin to directly reach the bloodstream. Pure essential oils can help in relieving a wide assortment of aches, pains, and injuries. They also act on the central nervous system. Thus pure essential oils as an alternative therapy for depression, anxiety, stress, relaxing and restoring emotional and physical well being.

Each essential oil has a different effect and can be used either alone or in combination to produce the desired effect. Different people have different reactions to the same aroma. A large amount of plant material is used to produce even a small amount of pure essential oils. For this reason, pure essential oils are expensive. Yet, only a few drops at one time are used to give the benefit.

The role of pure essential oils is indispensable in today's society. With the stress levels of people rising by the day, sadness, grief, anxiety, and depression are ever so common. With the increase in emotional imbalances, there are dramatic effects on the body as well. By choosing the right sort of pure essential oil you can experience an overall improvement in health. Incorporate pure essential oils as a part of your healthy lifestyle and add zest to your life today.

Made in the USA
Las Vegas, NV
06 December 2023